Inner Sanctum of Nursing And Rehab Care

WELCOME MESSAGE!

This book is being published as an educational tool and to give you information that is not found in general publications regarding what to look for when you or a relative needs nursing or rehab care. Most articles just tell you that you watch for cleanliness, odors, and do patients look clean and are they dressed. Most articles dwell on cleanliness and odors in a facility. I decided to write this HandBook after spending 26 days in a rehab facility because of a broken hip. During my 85 years of living, 17 years of my work experience was in social service agencies. Five of those were in a treatment Center for emotionally disturbed boys, 6-12 years of age. Twelve years was spent as Administrator of a 165 bed retirement and nursing home for the The American Lutheran Church, We were considered one of the best facilities in the State of Washington. After my discharge from rehab my conscious said I had to alert people to the many underlying bad care actions that went on and are covered up in many subtle ways. I do dwell a lot on the poor food service and an inadequate dietary department. This is on purpose because the food quality is poor to bad and good food and diet are necessary for your bones and muscles to build strength so you can go home.

This book will be boring to read, but can be a great benefit and resource to anyone looking for help to be admitted to a nursing or rehab care facility. The format will be in a diary format giving any reader a day by day blow. By doing this you can decide what you need to look for before you make any decision to admit yourself or a loved one to a facility. This book will give you a guide of what to look and listen for from your loved one.

COPYRIGHT

Dedication

This book is dedicated to my wonderful and lovely wife Giovanina and our daughter Deborah who was with her mother while I was in rehab. This book is also dedicated to all of our children who came to visit after I was discharged and to rest of our children, all our friends and relatives who kept us in their prayers.

Accolades!

To all the Professional Nurses, a few Nursing Aides, My Two PT Therapists and Cleaning Staff. You know who you are and my hat goes off to you because you care but are stymied by Administration staff that buries and ignores the many major complaints from your patients.

Definition of Term:

OT = Occupation Therapy

PT = Physical Therapy

Table Of Contents

Inner Sanctum of Nursing And Rehab Care

"ENTER THE INTERSANCTUM OF HELL"

Chapter 1 First Week of Hell!

Admission to this Rehab Facility was on the late afternoon of February 9, 2015 Admission was into a double patient room that was clean and no odor. After being settled in by the staff it was time for the supper hour,(which I will refer to as the light meal of the day) and lunch time was their heavy meal of the day. Supper consisted of (my choice) egg salad sandwich which was all egg white chopped in large peices with GOBS of mayonnaise. I took two bites and could not stand eating a gooey egg white salad sandwich.

I got settled to go to sleep and due to anxiety of moving from the hospital to a new setting I started to have chest, back-and shoulder pain. I reported the symptoms to a nursing aide. I gave her explicit information for her to have the charge nurse call my cardiologist's emergency service and report my symptoms and they would call the Doctor.

In a few minutes the Medicine Nurse came in and said —"take this-it is a pain pill" I refused the pill as the cardiologist had not approved the medicine. I said he would probably order a Nitro pill. Guess what? A nitro pill appeared in a matter of minutes which they had to take from their emergency medicine kit which all rehab centers have.

I knew no one called the Doctor but at moment I did not care as I wanted to get rid of the pain and after 15 minutes the little pill did its job. This whole scene was very poor professional nursing. #1.I am almost sure they did not call the Dr. because of the time span. # 2.They did not take my vital signs or listen to my heart beat. This is when I became aware that I was going to have to watch whatever came my way and plenty did over the coming days.

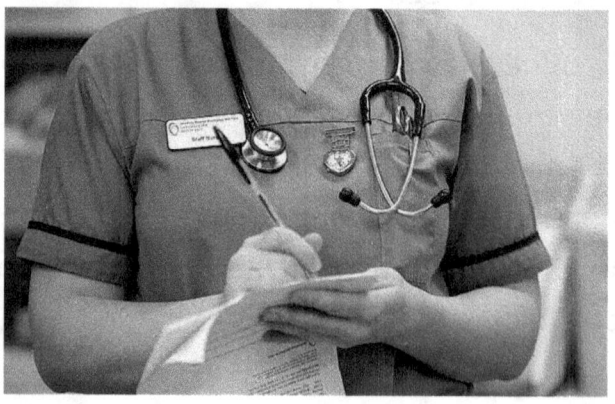

No Vital Signs

Woke up Tuesday morning 02/10/15 and was greeted with, a cold breakfast and "Where are your shorts as you have to get dressed for Physical Therapy." My question was "What shorts?" as I do not have any-and no one advised me or my wife what we were to bring. All I had was the few clothes that I went to the hospital with. They knew I was coming but no one bothered to call my wife and advise what clothes and supplies I would need. Also, their marketing staff person visited the hospital and knew I was to be admitted to rehab. She should have advised me or my wife what we were to bring. I did have clean underwear and T-shirts when I came from the hospital.

They found a pair of shorts and I went to change, sponge bathe myself and had to go to bathroom before I could go to therapy. The aides leave water running because they say keeps water warm for bathing and if you turn off it takes to long to get back to warm temperature. "What a Waste of Water!" I urinated and all at once my clothes were totally wet and thought the water had run over from the sink. Shut water off and they said they would call maintenance. So no clothes and went to PT in my clean knit boxer shorts and in hospital gown. This became a very embarrassing issue for me as it happened the next morning also. It was not the water overflowing, it was me urinating all over my clothes when sitting on the toilet.

I discovered the problem after I went to the bathroom again later. The appliance they were using to raise the toilet seat was an old rusty app that did not have the shield to direct your urine into the toilet bowl. There was a 2-3 inch crack between the app and the regular toilet bowl. At 85 you do not hang like you "usta" so unless you direct your private parts you are going to pee on yourself.

Finally, I made it to therapy after cleaning up and had my first PT session. After a brief rest here comes the OT Therapist. Her greeting is, "I am here to take you to OT for an evaluation." I said I do not need OT and the response was that they have to do this as Medicare requires it. I did not quite buy this as it has always been my perception that the Physician makes an order for any evaluation. But, I went along with it and was I ever surprised of what the evaluation consisted of. The initial assessment consisted of two and one half pages of treatment and goals that they did on their own because they bamboozled me with the Medicare requirement. I found out later this was against patient rights because all treatment for any therapy must come from a Doctor's order. They put their assessment together and then presented it to my physician two days after my admission and he signed it as being an order, On that first day in OT I spent no more than an hour doing a Barthal Modified Place Mat Test and received a grade of 98 per the therapist. How they came up with the assessment leaves many questions in my mind and what a great way to collect money for doing nothing. There notes also state that I had a hip replacement and I did not. I had a hip fracture

After returning to my room and visit with my wife a Nurse Aide comes in. It was change of shifts and said in a very aggressive voice. "I hear you refused to go to therapy today." I was shocked and told her she was nuts. I did not refuse to go to any therapy and I confirmed this with the PT Therapist who was present during the clothing situation. He confirmed that I did not do any such thing, The Day aide probably got ticked off because we complained that somebody should have let us know what clothes we were to bring, All was peaceful and ate their cold meal and was ready for the day to end.

Tuesday
February 10, 2015
Started with cold breakfast (the only thing hot is the coffee). OT therapist shows up and states she is there to take me to OT again. I said I am sorry

but I do not need OT and she insisted that they had to do more tests so I gave in. The test consisted of lifting a couple two pound weights which I did about 20 times and then running a gizmo that tension could be adjusted and was like bicycle pedals that you pumped up. I did this for about 10 minute s and that was the end. But according to the assessment record I would have to have been there for at least an hour and I was not. The rest of the day was with PT and then bed rest and visiting with family. My wonderful wife also brought me home cooked food so I would have decent meals while I was in rehab. Day went by until about Midnight and aide comes in and states she has to weigh me (At 11:00 PM?) So the scales put me at 130 lbs. which means I lost almost 25 lbs from 02/09/15 to 02/11/15. I remarked –How could that be? And the answer was that is what the scale states. OK and the rest of the day was put to rest until the next day.

Wednesday
February 11, 2015

During the day I was visited by the Admission Person-Dietary Dept. And Social Services, Dietary covered likes and dislikes. The dislikes were cooked spinach and iced Tea. Dietary also advised me that she noted my weight loss in the chart and thought that was too much weight to lose in couple days but did not question it. She then advised me that the orders stated that I was to be weighted daily for four straight days. Admissions brought in their welcome package which was three days late and had me sign the admitting papers, the Social Service person advised that we would have a planning care session on Friday 2/13/15.

Thursday AM
02/12/15
The Day started with a cold breakfast. Cold over cooked omelet, cold dry biscuit OJ and only hot thing on tray (hot coffee.) The food carts set in the hallway for over 1/2 hour before food was served. You learn quickly that if you complain about cold food their answer is always,"we will heat it up for you" and you do not micro wave over cooked eggs and biscuits as you have rubber eggs and a wet soggy biscuit. Any professional chef will tell you, do not use a micro wave to warm or heat up certain foods and eggs and bread are products you do not warm up.
The day after breakfast started with OT again. After two short sessions previous to this day I said no more to myself. This OT is what I refer to as a young college student who acts like a scared teenager trying to smile like she is so confident.

You are treated like a teenager as they act like they are scared to death of an old man.. They start with I am so and so and before we go to OT I need to ask you some questions. This is between their embarrassing little giggle Tee Hee's and they start with Birthday –what is your occupation and the I stopped them right there with, "I am not answering any of your questions."- Go back to my chart and you will find all your answers and do your homework and if you are trying to prove that I am nuts then you better try something else. If you want to know if you are talking to the right person , then check my wrist band that has all the info and I am not doing a dog and pony show for you and then I send them out.

After a time my favorite people show for my PT appointment and we proceed with the exercises they have set up for me. The PT department has an excellent staff except for one person who is so lazy he does nothing to promote good recovery exercise and the PT Supervisor is lax in making sure you are covered for your appointment if a therapist does not come to work, and does not keep up with physician orders. I will cover this later on in another chapter.

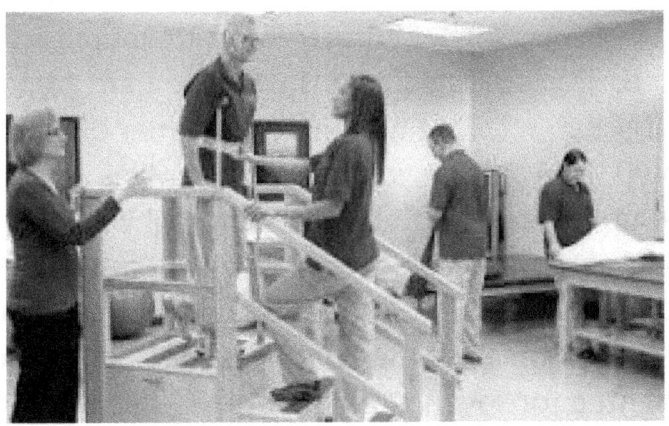

Great Therapy Session

Lunch and dinner were provided by my wife with home cooked food so was a great day at the table. This day ended on a good note except for OT' harassment.

Friday
February 13, 2015
Breakfast was cold pancakes, overcooked cold scrambled eggs, and hot cereal was cold.
Then the visits start with OT. The Tee Hee's are back wanting same information and I tell them again, I am not going to OT and any info get it off my chart and they left- The next appointment was PT and another good session getting to where I could almost get out of bed on my own but still needed a little help to lift my right leg off the bed to get into wheel chair. In the afternoon we had our planning care conference which was managed

by the Social Service Director who announced she makes all plans and decides when you are going to be discharged. That was the eye opener of what would be in store if you bucked her plans. She definitely does not fit the definition of what a Social service person does. My weight loss was brought up and they agreed that was not right so the head nurse put me on orders that I would be weighted for seven straight days. PT said I would be there for at least 4 weeks and he was right on. They asked if we had any any complaints, and yes we did. Keep OT out of the treatment loop because I did not need OT. Made the complaint about cold food and same old answer (we can heat it up for you.) I actually laughed and told them you do not heat up the food you serve because it is the kind of food you destroy when you put it in the micro wave. I told them to watch a few professional TV cooking shows and you will learn a Micro Wave is not the cure for warming food. I said I did not like my hot cereal being cold when its gets to you and then when you add cold milk you get very cold hot cereal.

 Rest of day was visits with my wife and daughter. They brought me my lunch and dinner for the next two days. Rest of the day after my luscious homemade dinner, was TV, rest and relax. Later in the night came the new weigh in schedule after missing two nights of the first four days because no one read the orders. On a new scale device I weighed in at 150 lbs. Called it a night.

Saturday
February 14, 2015
Breakfast was served barely warm sausage gravy and undercooked biscuit which was still doughy inside plus their overcooked rubber scrambled eggs. This is where it gets interesting and the cover up of your complaints start. With your food tray you get a printed note that has a few notes etc on it to remind the servers what not to put on your tray.. My note now has new information which is the next day after my complaints at the planning session. My previous sheets did not have any complaints and now I have as follows: Dislikes-Cereal-Liver, Milk, Spinach and Tea. Now remember what I said at the meeting-"hot cereal is cold when it arrives, put cold milk on the so called hot cereal. and it gets colder, not sure where spinach comes from but OK because I do not like spinach and I said Iced Tea and they put down tea, but I do drink hot tea, and **I did not say I disliked milk** and there was not any discussion about liver. This is all documented because I saved all my daily dietary notes. I Finished the day with weigh in at 150 +lbs.

Chapter 2   Second Week Of Pandemonium!

Sunday
February 15, 2015

Was a quiet day, breakfast was cold overcooked potatoes and rubber scrambled eggs and served on a cool plate. I did my own PT exercises. The day passed quietly except for anther visit by a week end OT person and refused to participate. Went for weigh in at 11:30 PM and I am still bewildered why the weigh ins have to be around midnight.

Monday
February 16, 2015
They woke me to go for weigh in at 12:30 AM. After weigh in and back to my room. I asked aide to get me two extra strength Tylenol from med nurse as needed to cover pain so I could sleep rest of the night. The aide got all flustered and said I should have asked for the Tylenol as we were coming back from weigh in as we went right by the med cart. There was not a med nurse in sight except a nurse was on the phone. That is all I knew. The aide was indignant that she had to go a few feet and ask the med nurse to bring me the Tylenol. The aide gave the nurse the wrong information and just told her that I needed a pain

pill. So after a short time the nurse brings me a Tramadol which is the stronger pain med.to take depending on my pain level. When I got the pill I just said I ordered Tylenol but just give me the damn pill as someone can't fulfill a simple request without getting bent out of shape.   **"Very Unprofessional"**

Tuesday
February 17, 2015

Breakfast was cool served on a cold plate. Over cooked scrambled eggs like rubber, cold corn beef hash and a doughy unbaked roll. Hottest thing on the tray was coffee. Rest of day had my PT schedule and OT stayed away and night went well.

Wednesday Thursday

February 18-19, 2015

Both of these days went pretty good except for the food. Breakfast on Wednesday was cold French Toast cold scrambled Eggs, Sausage cold. Plate was cold and coffee was just warm. They missed weight schedule.

Thursday breakfast the biscuits were soggy, plate not even warm, Passed on rest of meals except for fruit and dinner was my home cooked meals

Friday

February 20. 2015

Breakfast was lousy as usual, cold or lukewarm with tough pancakes, cold eggs, cold bacon and plate was cold. Lunch was over cooked fish, under cooked carrots and cold. Had regular PT session which are always good because they do their job and do it well, Decided to have lunch to give my wife a break and lunch was same as rest of dietary meals. LOUSY! .

About 5:00 PM I put in a request for 2 ES Tylenol. 2nd request went at 1:45 AM on 02/21/15. Third request was at 4:20 AM. And after 4th reminder the request was fulfilled at 4:40 AM.

IS THIS WHAT YOU CALL GOOD NURSING CARE ACCORDING TO THEIR BROCHURES?

Saturday

February 21, 2015!

Saturday already started on a bad note with the goof on medicine. So here we go with the gourmet meals that are really not meals but glorified garbage. Breakfast was biscuits with sausage gravy and eggs. (One of My Favorites) This meal was ruined by under baked biscuits (doughy inside) cold gravy, cold plate and cold eggs. Biscuits are to be golden brown when baked properly and the biscuits hardly had a tan color to them. To give my wife a break I chose to do dinner and what a disaster. Pulled pork is meat that is pulled into strips and this pulled pork had to be run through a food processor because it was just plain mush. Corn Fritters were not done and corn in the fritters was soft and not cooked. The best on the menu were the baked beans if they had been even warm but they were cold and the plate was cold,

For some reason they did not take my vital signs on this day.

Chapter 3-Third Week of A Confused OT Department

Sunday
February 22, 2015

This week started out OK with the usual cold breakfast, cold plate and corned beef hash as a filling for the overcooked omelet. So what is new.. Later in the morning here comes the substitute OT with the song and dance that I had to show I could stand in front of a mirror and shave myself, could I get to bathroom with the walker and could I sponge bathe myself and put my clothes on. I was already dressed and no one helped me and by this time I could get out of bed with help with my leg on the injured hip side. I politely told her in a very loud voice to get the hell out of my room and I was not putting on any dog and pony show for any OT. Secondly I do not shave as I use an electric shaver and you do not need a mirror to shave with an electric razor. Also, she did not read any records because I had been using a walker and tending to myself. During the day I did my own exercising walking in the halls with my walker,

I ate their dinner and supper to give my wife another break. Another disaster which was a cheese burger on a cold plate and bun was damp and soggy as they put the cheese on the bottom layer. Cheese is never on the bottom. The rest of the day was OK and uneventful. The day closed with aides taking my vitals and giving me my weigh in.

Monday

February 23, 2015

Uneventful day with usual cold breakfast but this one had a new twist with pancakes that were cold and they had a hard crust ring around the pancake that was so tough you could hardly cut with a fork. I showed the aide and she just shrugged her shoulders and walked out. They know their dietary department is a lost cause and you sure do not see them eating any meals. We have asked several of the employees if they eat the food and they all look at you like you are crazy.

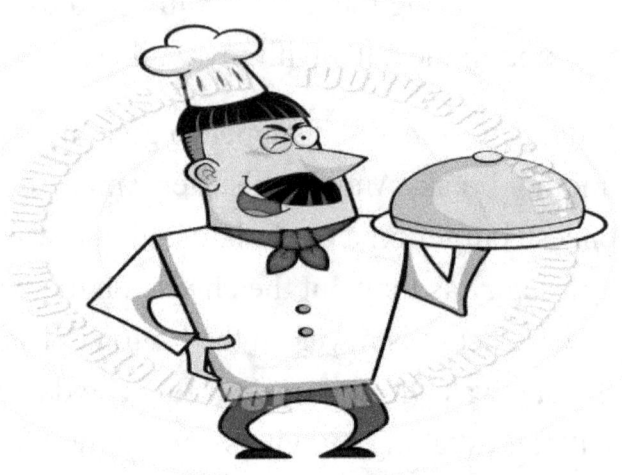

They Should Employ A Professional Chef!

Food Manager & Dietary Staff!

At 2 PM PT therapist did not show for my appointment, An aide from OT showed up at 3 PM under the guise that I was going to PT. As we were going to the appointment I asked, are we going to PT and she said no, that she was taking me to OT. I said you are not taking me to OT. I told her that I have requested several times there will not be any OT. I refused 3 times on Sunday 02/22/15 and at least five times previous to today. They had to see if I could take care of myself and I said read the chart. I go to the bathroom, I wash myself, and if I had rubber arms I could wash my back (only help I needed). I need PT to strengthen my legs and hip so I can walk normally with a walker, then a cane and then natural. I can get along at home and I have the proper equipment at home.

Lunch was another disaster with chicken salad sandwich on wet damp white bread. The macaroni salad was dry and the chicken salad on the sandwich was so thin that you were actually eating only bread. You wondered where the chicken flew off to.

They finished the day with Vitals and they weighed me.

Tuesday and Wednesday

February 24, 25, 2015

Breakfast was cold-plate was cold-cold rubber eggs-salty overcooked corned beef hash (I think they have stock in the Corned beef hash company as they serve it so much.) and a small breakfast roll.

My primary physician came to see me, at my request as Tuesday is his day to visit the facility. He is also the house physician. I told him that he had to put in an order to stop OT staff from coming and insisting I had to go to OT sessions. Also, add to the order that I was to receive PT twice a day, Monday Through Saturday and a PT to supervise my walking exercise on Sunday. The order was executed and the new schedule was to be effective February 23, 2015.

Day ended with vitals and sleep.

Wednesday was same kind of day with cold breakfast,, PT sessions. Today was to remove staples which meant that I could have and take a shower. The day passed with night time vitals but no weigh in.

February 26, 2015

Thursday

Same cold breakfast, just different food. Have not received a shower even though I asked and the request was ignored. I caught an aide and asked her when I would get a shower and she informed me that my shower days were Wednesday and Friday. Now this is Thursday so my day was missed without any explanation, I went for my two PT sessions and then an OT showed up to go to OT again, and I told her to leave and asked a nurse that I wanted to see the Social Service Director today. She came to my room in a little while. I told her that I was going to raise hell with someone if they did not get OT off my back. She backed down from her attitude that she makes all planning care decisions and said that I would have to take this up with the Therapy Manager. She left, and the Therapy Manager came in and I had to tell her to back off with OT. She went into the excuse that I needed this and had to have it so I could take care of myself when I got home. I informed her that if another OT showed up she was going against Doctors orders. She said what orders so that meant she did not check any doctor's orders from Tuesday Morning until Thursday afternoon.. Admitting she was not aware of the new orders. She left to check. She came back with a PT therapist and said new orders would be carried out. I also became aware that this is set up to get more OT billing hours for clients, Medicare and insurance companies. If you are getting something you do not need, do not let them do anything unless you have a doctor's order. They are lining their pockets with $$$$, billing for services not needed and in my case billing for services not performed nor ordered. They cover themselves by looking like they are doing an assessment. Then they have a physician sign the paperwork after the fact to make it look like he or she made the order. I know this happens because it happened to me. I confirmed this with my Doctor that he signed the OT assessment order and he did not order an assessment. His original order was for PT only. They placed their assessment in front of him and he just automatically signed off on it. His answer was of course- you have to talk to the facility. .Yes, I will be talking to the facility about this, but not directly. When this book is published I am going to take this whole scene to higher authorities such as Medicare and my insurance company. **Do not forget that by law you have patient rights. Memorize or acquaint yourself with the major ones.**

 The rest of the day passed with vitals and the night weigh in. Asked aide to be weighed at 12;30 PM and they came at 5:15 PM.

February27, 2015

Friday

My wife and daughter took a break because they wanted to do some shopping so took on the dietary meals for the day. It was a riot. Breakfast was cold, plate was cold, eggs were like rubber and pancakes were cold and tough. I ate the eggs just to have something on my stomach. During the day I went to my double PT sessions,

Lunch was undercooked fish that was soggy and wet in the middle. Peas ere dry cold and no liquid in the dish and very bland without any seasoning, French Fries were cold and like eating rubber sticks.

The evening meal was roast beef sandwich on white bread. The beef was over cooked and tough. The plate and sandwich were ice cold and they had to have been in the refrigerator for at least two hours. They were served with corned beef hash and overcooked onion rings. The hash and onion rings were on the ice cold plate but were supposed to be hot. The onion rings were like chewing on rubber bands. I complained to the nurse and she said that sandwiches are supposed to be served cold.

This shows you how little the aides are taught about dietary standards. Any person that does any cooking knows you do not put hot food on an ice cold plate. The dietary standard is that hot foods that accompany cold food is to be put in separate warm containers to maintain a temperature of 115 Degrees when the food reaches the patient..

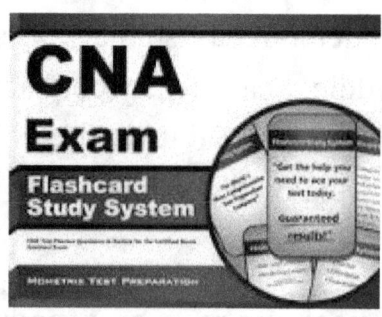

Educate Your Staff Instead Of Them

Giving Patients Stupid Answers!

February 28, 2015

Saturday

Breakfast was cold sausage gravy on a biscuit that was done but the cold gravy shot the biscuit down the tube. The eggs were like rubber and cold but ate them just to have some food in my body.

One PT session was missed by manager as she did not schedule a replacement PT for my regular PT was only available for one session. However, the assessment sheet shows I had two treatments. I did an extra walk exercise on my own to make up for the missed PT appointment.

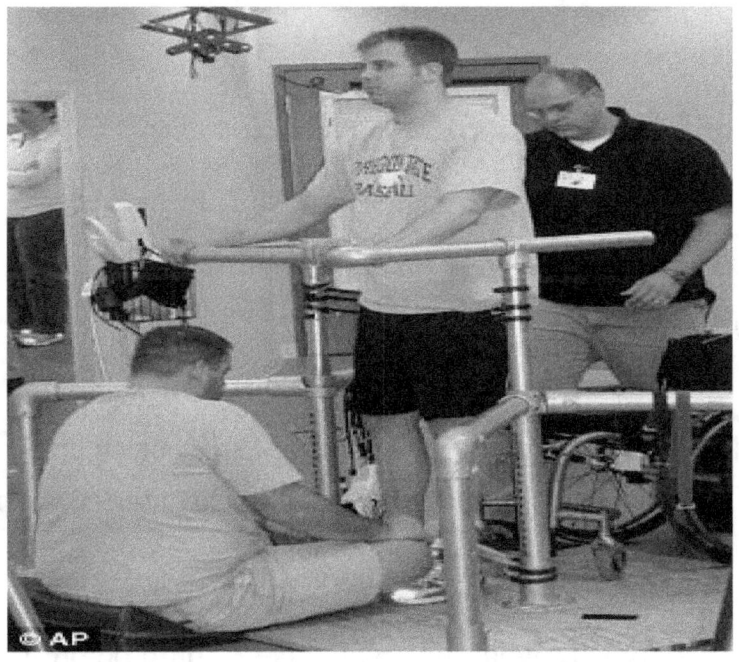

They Have Good PT Therapists & Equipment!

No shower and was skipped over again. I finished the day with dinner from home, rested and slept the night through.

Sunday

March 1, 2015

Days were drawing to a close as only had six more days per the Physical Therapy Department. Then I would be going home. The Day started with usual cold breakfast. I convinced the charge .nurse that I was going to have a shower today or else. Was not sure what the "what else" would be but I would have thought up something because this had become totally out of control for good nursing care.

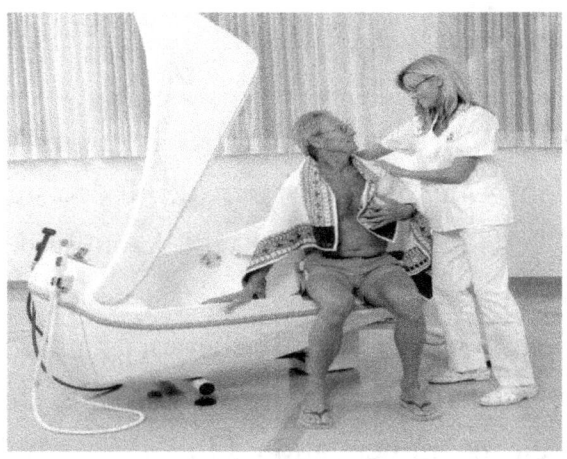

What A Great Feeling After 20 Plus Days Of Sponge Baths!

No PT Therapist (even though he walked by my room several times) showed up so did my own walking the halls seven times during the day.

March 2, 2015

Monday

Rest of the day was usual routine-cold meals-PT exercises and my wife came to visit. Then the surprise came while she was visiting as the Social Service Director came to the room to advise us that I would be going home on March 13th and not March 7, 2015. I asked who made that decision and her answer was, "I Do as I make all plans for patients discharge. I asked what happened to the PT Department stating I could go home on March 7. She informed us that she made all decisions and I said like Hell you do and I will be out of here on March 7, come hell or high water. She left, and I immediately went to my PT therapists and asked them what changed and they said nothing changed from their recommendation. I told them that if I was not discharged on March 7th they would have the biggest dog and pony show in the front of their facility as I would call the sheriff office, local TV Channels and tell them I was being held against my will. Then via the grapevine I found out that this was a ploy to get more days for billing.

I had a Dr.visit with my orthopedic surgeon and advised him of the situation. He said that they cannot keep you against your will and if you want to leave, you just have to have someone pick you up.

The word from the PT Department must have gotten to the Social Service Director. When I got back to my room there was a discharge form on my night stand that said I would be discharged on March 7.

Also, a statement that equipment for home use would be delivered to my room before I went home.(I put this here for a reason which will be referred to later on discharge day.)

March 03 through March 07, 2015

Tuesday Through Saturday (Discharge Day)

During this week an incident happened that is unbelievable to the extent of what some employees will do to cover up their mistakes of mishandling a patient. A 90 plus year old man, (mentally confused) was admitted and was in the bed next to mine. He came from Arkansas because he broke his hip and could not care for himself and he needed rehab. His daughter (living in Florida) admitted him. As soon as she admitted her father I could tell by her expressions that this was tearing her apart. Because of my experience I asked her about her father and told her that this would be very hard for her emotionally and just take a day at a time and understand that he does not know what he is doing and does not have any clue that he is verbally striking out at you, and does not recognize you most of the time. Hopefully I helped her. Her father still thought he was in Arkansas. One evening two aides came bouncing into the room and in very demanding bully voices," we are taking you for a shower as this is your shower day. (I wish someone would have told me that.) and immediately he said no you are not and I am not going. They argued with him some more and he kept saying no and more they argued the more belligerent he became. They finally got him in a wheel chair and they went to the shower.

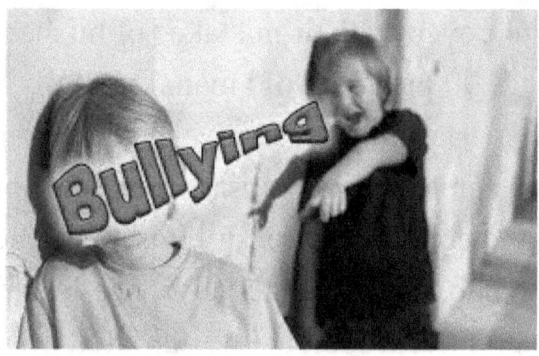

Later in the evening they came in again with same bullying demanding voices that they were going to put him in bed for the night. He refused and told them he was not going to bed. I did not see what happened but heard the conversation. It was apparent that they were forcing him into bed and he got belligerent and grabbed one of the aides and she said in a very loud voice, "let go of my arm, you are hurting me.' They left and you could tell they were disgusted. The next morning a Sheriff's deputy showed up with the Administrator and they looked into his side of the room. They left without any comment. Later the daughter came in and I asked her what happened and she said the aides accused her father of sexual assault. This was so farfetched and bold lies. The two aides outweighed her father by at least 150 # and he was so weak you could push him over with a toothpick.

The facility waited 17 hours before they contacted the daughter and then threatened her, that she should probably move her father because he was not the type patient they wanted. This was pure hogwash because over half their patients are confused. As I pointed out previously, they need to train their aides how to work with patients. It is interesting to note that the next night the nurse came on duty and because she knew her stuff she handled the patient all by herself, did not need any help and all went well because of her approach to patient care.

I watched carefully on Friday to see if the toilet appliance would arrive and it did not. The Social Service Director after her great speech d of, (she takes care of everything did not check to see if the appliance arrived in my room. On Saturday before it came time to leave I advised the head nurse that the appliance was not there and showed her the order. She stated that appliances are always delivered to the patient's home. She tried several calls and she could not make contact with the appliance company or the Social Worker. She took it upon herself to scrounge in their house equipment and found a new appliance in a storage unit. We loaded this in our car and we were out of there. I was free and could go home to in home nursing care and PT.

One last note: You remember I said earlier I was to be weighed for seven straight days. I did a count as kept track and it took them 14 days to do seven straight days. **(Great Way To Follow Orders)**

SUMMARY OF THE REHAB CARE!

`Some of the readers may want to just read this summary. However I would suggest reading the book in its entirety to know what you should be looking for even if you decide to admit yourself or a loved one.

No.1. Check for a clean facility and no odors or very little.

No.2. Visit at meal time so you can observe how food is handled and look at the trays to see if the food is presented in an appealing manner.

No.3. Ask pointed questions and see if there is any hesitation in answers. If there is any hesitation or I can't answer, look deeper and prod until you get an answer.

No. 4 .Check out other patients and see if they are dressed and not in hospital gowns unless they are bedridden.

No.5. If you admit someone, listen to what they are telling you. Then check it out. For example, if they complain about the food bring in a cell phone camera and take pictures. Use a needle thermometer and check the temp of the food when it arrives at bedside or in the room. Hot food temps are to be at 115 Degrees when food arrives to the patent..

Remember that every time they are delivering a meal to patients under their present system they are breaking the law and not meeting state or

federal facility requirements. Request the medical records to make sure they have Dr. Orders to do what they are doing and if nursing notes are being followed..

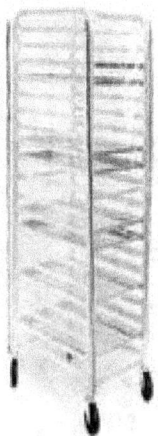

This Is Their Antique Tray Delivery System!

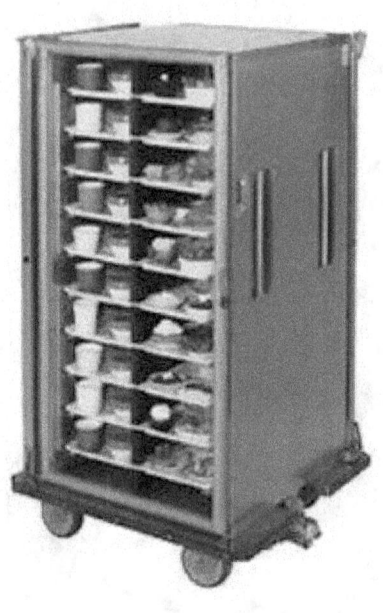

This Is The Modern Day Food Delivery System
With Hot and Cold Partitions. Has Been Available
Since Early 1970's!